REKINDLING INTIMACY AND PASSION IN YOUR MARRIAGE

Pst Harrison Okechukwu E

ISBN:9798337531250

Cover design by: Art Painter
Library of Congress Control Number: 2018675309
Printed in the United States of America

Dedicated to every marriage that nearly shipwrecked,
but survived by the grace of God.

CONTENTS

INTRODUCTION

A user's manual typically accompanies every mechanical or electrical appliance purchased. It is the manufacturer's guide, designed to educate the user on how to properly operate and maintain the machine. In the same way, we cannot effectively address the issues affecting the institution of marriage without first examining its origin, purpose, and principles for application.

While there are scientific theories surrounding man's origin, tradition, myth, and religion all converge on a singular truth—that marriage is as old as humanity itself. This affirms the doctrine of creation. Most traditions and religions agree that the human race originated from one man and one woman—Adam and Eve—whom God created as the first human beings.

"Then God said, 'Let Us make man in Our image, according to Our likeness; let them have dominion over the fish of the sea, over the birds of the air, and over the cattle, over all the earth and over every creeping thing that creeps on the earth.'" Genesis 1:26, NKJV

"Then the Lord God formed the man from the dust of the ground. He breathed the breath of life into the man's nostrils, and the man became a living person." Genesis 2:7, NLT

Upon creating man, God saw that it was not good for him to be alone. Hence, He created a helper—a companion uniquely suited for him.

"Then the Lord God said, 'It is not good for the man to be alone. I will make a helper who is just right for him.'" Genesis 2:18, NLT

Understanding the purpose and foundation of marriage requires us to return to the Manufacturer's Manual—the Word of God. Only through His lens can we rightly interpret the value, function, and transformative power of marriage.

ACKNOWLEDGEMENT

I am deeply indebted to everyone whose work, both online and offline, along with their wealth of experience, significantly impacted me during the development of this book. Special thanks to my beloved wife, Mrs. Harrison Jemimah Nkem, who believed in the grace of God upon my life and supported me in every possible way. Nne, may God richly bless you.

To all the married couples who allowed me to counsel them during difficult moments in their marriages—for which, by God's grace, solutions were found and restoration occurred—I say thank you. May your marriages continue to grow in strength and grace.

To everyone who made a meaningful impact on this journey using their time, wisdom, and resources, may the Lord, who never forgets any labor of love, reward you immensely.

PREFACE

Marriage is a profound, rich, and complex institution that has stood as the cornerstone of human society for centuries. It is a sacred journey between a consenting adult male and female, united in love, trust, and mutual support. This book, Rekindling Intimacy and Passion in Your Marriage, is an intimate exploration of the human experience within this divine union—delving into its joys, its challenges, and its transformative power.

Here, we examine the multifaceted aspects of marriage: from its cultural and historical contexts to its emotional and psychological dimensions. We reflect on how marriage transforms—and is transformed by—the individuals within it, their communities, and the society at large.

This work is dedicated to unveiling the beauty and complexity of marriage, acknowledging both its triumphs and its trials. By shedding light on the realities of married life, we aim to cultivate empathy, appreciation, and support for those navigating this remarkable journey.

While many books on marriage and family exist, too often they offer solutions to surface-level problems without addressing the deeper wounds or foundational issues threatening this sacred institution. This book is not just another title to fill a bookshelf; it is a heartfelt guide for rekindling the lost intimacy and passion within your marriage.

Getting the foundation right is key. As the Bible declares, "If the foundation be destroyed, what can the righteous do?" (Psalm

11:3). Sadly, modernity disguised as civilization has eroded the core values our forebears left for us. If the family unit is this fragile in our time, what hope remains for future generations?

Divorce rates are increasingly alarming. Families are torn apart, lives hurt, and the emotional toll often falls heaviest on the children—products of once-promising unions. In Africa and many parts of the world, the definition and purpose of marriage have been misunderstood. Until we return to the true essence of marriage as designed by its Originator—God—the problems plaguing this divine institution will persist.

May the truths and insights within this book bring healing, renewal, and strength to your marriage, and inspire you to see this institution not through the lens of culture or modern trends, but through the eternal eyes of its Creator.

CHAPTER 1:

The Purpose of the Marriage Institution

1. Originator's Intention – God's View

In Genesis 2:18, God identified a critical need in Adam—not a physical or material need, but a psychological one. Though Adam was physically sound and productively engaged:

"Then the Lord God placed the man in the Garden of Eden to tend and watch over it." Genesis 2:15, NLT

He lacked emotional connectivity, relational intimacy, and companionship. God said:

"It is not good for the man to be alone..." Genesis 2:18, NKJV

Loneliness, when left unaddressed, destabilizes emotional well-being, often leading to frustration, depression, and unhealthy behaviors such as addiction or promiscuity. According to Longman Dictionary, loneliness is "a state of being unhappy because you are alone or do not have anyone to talk to." Merriam-Webster defines it as "sad from being alone" or "producing a feeling of bleakness."

It's important to distinguish between being alone and being lonely. Solitude can be refreshing and necessary—for prayer, meditation, and self-reflection:

"As He was alone praying, His disciples joined Him." Luke 9:18, NKJV

"Then Jacob was left alone; and a man wrestled with him until the breaking of day." Genesis 32:24, NKJV

Yet loneliness, as Evangelist Billy Graham once observed, "is the feeling of emptiness on the inside, that though in the midst of a crowd, one still feels isolated."

Loneliness is not confined to singles—it can afflict married individuals, urban dwellers, or the elite, especially in a society where "every man lives to himself." Emotional disconnection is the breeding ground for loneliness.

"I am like an owl in the desert, like a little owl in a far-off wilderness. I lie awake, lonely as a solitary bird on the roof." Psalm 102:6–7, NLT

Understanding this helps us appreciate Genesis 2:18 more deeply. God, in His omniscience, saw the emotional void in Adam and provided a divine solution:

"I will make him a helper suitable for him." Genesis 2:18, LB

Marriage was not man's invention—it was God's. He carefully designed it and handed it to man as a divine trust. Therefore, we must consult God's Word to understand His intentions.

Many hold skewed perceptions of marriage. Some believe it exists primarily for:

- ❖ Procreation
- ❖ Sexual gratification
- ❖ Proving maturity or responsibility

While these are functions of marriage, they are not its original purpose. The foundational reason is clearly spelled out in Genesis 2:18: companionship and partnership.

God never intended marriage to be a master-servant arrangement, but a mutual partnership where both husband and wife are stakeholders. It was only after the fall that the dynamics changed:

"You will desire to control your husband, but he will rule over you." Genesis 3:16, NLT

"But I want you to understand that the head of every man is Christ, the head of a woman is man, and the head of Christ is God." 1 Corinthians 11:3, NKJV

The prevalent struggles in marriage today often stem from misconceptions. While procreation is God's expectation, it is not His purpose. Let's revisit:

"Then God blessed them, and God said to them, 'Be fruitful and multiply; fill the earth and subdue it...'" Genesis 1:28, NKJV

This passage does not define the purpose of marriage, but reveals God's empowerment for human flourishing. The phrase "God blessed them" (Hebrew: Barak) signifies divine empowerment— God equipping the couple to thrive emotionally, spiritually, and relationally.

God's real focus is found in Genesis 2:18 and consummated in verses 21–25:

"So the Lord God caused the man to fall into a deep sleep... Then the Lord God made a woman from the rib, and He brought her to the man... 'At last!' the man exclaimed. 'This one is bone from my bone, and flesh from my flesh!...'" Genesis 2:21–25, NLT

This was not a casual union—it was the blueprint of companionship and oneness. Without building marriage on these divine foundations, problems are inevitable.

The Three C's of a Thriving Marriage

To foster a happy and healthy marriage, couples must focus on three foundational pillars:

1. Companionship – Emotional closeness and mutual support.

2. Commitment – A steadfast decision to remain faithful and present.

3. Communication – Honest, open dialogue that nurtures

understanding.

Companionship:

Companionship is defined as "being with someone you enjoy being with and not being alone." The phrase "enjoy being with" implies that not everyone's presence brings joy. There are some individuals, despite their efforts to impress, whose presence you simply cannot enjoy—there's no bond, no ease, and certainly no friendship.

Marriage, at its very core, is a relationship built on friendship. This was the most fundamental need God observed in Adam. Though Adam had been appointed as the chief custodian of Earth and had abundant material resources at his disposal, something vital was still missing.

"Then the Lord God took the man and put him in the Garden of Eden to tend and keep it." Genesis 2:15–16, NKJV

Despite his responsibilities and blessings, Adam had a deep yearning for relationship—someone to talk to, laugh with, and emotionally connect with. God saw this emotional void and responded:

"And the Lord God said, 'It is not good that man should be alone; I will make him a helper comparable to him.'" Genesis 2:18, NKJV

In a survey I conducted years ago among both men and women, "companionship" emerged as the number one desire in marriage. No one wants to spend their life with a person who feels like a stranger—or worse, a "monster." Everyone longs to share life with a friend.

The best and closest friend every married person should have is their spouse. Marriage thrives when companionship is treasured.

"Enjoy life with the wife whom you love all the days of your fleeting life which He has given you under the sun—for this is your reward in life and in your toil in which you have labored under the sun." Ecclesiastes 9:9, NKJV

If your spouse's presence starts to irritate you, something has gone wrong. Bitterness may be growing, and love may be waning. In such moments, it's essential to realign your heart and prioritize your spouse again.

"This is my beloved, and this is my friend." Song of Solomon 5:16, NKJV

Commitment:

Commitment is defined as "a determination to keep the promise of doing something, or to behave in a particular way." It is also "an instance of being obligated or emotionally driven toward a cause or person."

Take the example of Chrissie Redden, a Canadian mountain biker who gave up a promising senior management career to train for the 2000 Olympics. When someone asked why athletes sacrifice so much for a single gold medal, the answer was simple: because it's worth it.

Likewise, your marriage is your gold medal event. It requires a double-layered commitment:

- ❖ A commitment to do what builds the relationship

- ❖ A commitment to avoid what weakens or threatens it

Marriage is not just about adding helpful elements (like love, romance, and communication); it's also about removing harmful ones—like pride, addiction, emotional neglect, or inappropriate friendships.

"For bodily exercise profits a little, but godliness is profitable for all things…" 1 Timothy 4:8, NKJV

"But solid food belongs to those who are of full age, that is, those who by reason of use have their senses exercised to discern both good and evil." Hebrews 5:14, NKJV

Ask yourself:

    a. What one thing could I stop doing today that would

improve my marriage?

Maybe it's a habit, an attitude, or a toxic relationship. Whatever it is, commit to releasing it.

"Throw off your old evil nature and your former way of life, which is rotten through and through, full of lust and deception. Instead, there must be a spiritual renewal of your thoughts and attitudes... Get rid of all bitterness, rage, anger, harsh words, and slander... Be kind to each other, tenderhearted, forgiving one another, just as God through Christ has forgiven you." Ephesians 4:22–32, NLT (selected)

Consider these reflection questions:

i].   Is my spouse emotionally troubled by how much attention I give to others or to work, media, or hobbies?

ii].   Am I emotionally or physically more intimate with someone else than with my spouse?

iii].   Does my spouse feel sidelined by my relationships with parents, siblings, or friends?

iv].   Is my spouse uncomfortable with my habits or behavior?

Marital commitment is the willingness to sacrifice your own needs to meet your spouse's needs, with the goal of building one another up in love.

"Under His direction, the whole body is fitted together perfectly. As each part does its own special work, it helps the other parts grow, so that the whole body is healthy and growing and full of love." Ephesians 4:16, NLT

Here are a few things to refrain from for the sake of your marriage:

- Emotional connections your spouse perceives as inappropriate

- Flirtation. "Do you not know that he who is joined to a harlot is one body with her?" — 1 Corinthians 6:16

- Addictive or destructive habits like smoking, drinking, or drug abuse, "All things are lawful… but not all things are helpful." — 1 Corinthians 6:12

- Being inconsistent in your words and actions, "Speaking the truth in love…" — Ephesians 4:15

- Harboring bitterness, temper, and conflict, "…forgive as the Lord forgave you." — Colossians 3:13

- Emotional insensitivity, "Husbands… be considerate… treat them with respect…" — 1 Peter 3:7

Breaking old habits is never easy, but it is essential for growth.

"I press on to possess that perfection for which Christ Jesus first possessed me… Forgetting the past and looking forward to what lies ahead, I press on to reach the end of the race and receive the heavenly prize…" Philippians 3:12–14, NLT

When companionship and communication are strained, commitment will carry you through. Like God's love for His people, your vow must endure.

"The Lord did not set His affection on you… because you were more numerous… but it was because the Lord loved you and kept the oath He swore…" Deuteronomy 7:7–9, NKJV

Three Principles of Commitment from Deuteronomy 7:7–9:

1. Set your affection on your spouse

2. Keep the oath you made at your wedding

3. Be faithful to your covenant of love

Communication:

Communication is defined as "the process of exchanging information or expressing your feelings, thoughts, and aspirations in a way that is understood by the other party." It also refers to the "interchange of thoughts or opinions through shared symbols or dialogue."

Communication is essential to human existence. Imagine a world where all forms of communication—verbal, written, nonverbal—are cut off. Life would become not only boring but chaotic. People would be unable to express themselves or relate with others. No one can read minds; therefore, it is only through communication that thoughts and intentions are known and understood.

God endowed mankind with the gift of communication so that we could share our thoughts, needs, emotions, and desires. Whenever there is a crisis in marriage—or in any relationship—it often points to one thing: a breakdown in communication. As the saying goes, "When jaw-jaw ends, war-war begins."

Sadly, many married couples hardly communicate beyond the necessities. They may live in the same house and sleep in the same bed, yet remain emotionally disconnected—strange bedfellows. Their interaction is limited to functional demands, such as financial needs or sexual intimacy. They miss out on true soul-connection, which only comes through intentional and transparent communication.

Reflection Questions:

1. How would you assess the quality of communication between you and your spouse?

2. Are there areas in your relationship where communication feels restricted?

3. Do you feel emotionally connected after sharing honest conversations?

4. What plans do you have to improve your communication?

Meaningful communication builds bridges. It reveals hidden dangers and heals emotional wounds. It must go deeper than surface-level conversation, like what happens between coworkers or staff. Spousal communication should be intimate, expressive, emotional, and complete.

A healthy marriage must foster a "no-holds-barred" approach—no restricted areas. Couples should be free to talk about everything: their past, future, finances, children, career, sex life, goals, and spiritual concerns.

When you feel unable to express yourself, anger and bitterness begin to fester. Bottled-up emotions can lead to emotional outbursts or silent vengeance. Genesis 2:25 offers a divine model of openness:

"And they were both naked, the man and his wife, and were not ashamed." Genesis 2:25, NKJV

This verse symbolizes complete transparency and vulnerability. They had no secrets, no pretense, no manipulation. They were open about their earnings, opinions, and emotions. They did not use sex as a weapon of control or punishment.

Statements like "I can't let my wife know how much I earn" or "I'll continue to use sex to punish him" reflect emotional immaturity. A person who withholds communication is not yet ready for marriage.

"Therefore, putting away lying, 'Let each one of you speak truth with his neighbor,' for we are members of one another." Ephesians 4:25, NKJV

"The husband should fulfill his wife's sexual needs, and the wife should fulfill her husband's needs. The wife gives authority over her body to her husband, and the husband gives authority over his body to his wife… so that Satan won't be able to tempt you because of your lack of self-control." 1 Corinthians 7:3–5, NLT

The Roots of Communication: Communion and Common:

Two key words help us understand the depth of marital communication: Communion and Common.

A. Communion

Communion means "sharing deeply with someone you feel

emotionally connected to." It involves fellowship, which goes beyond just physical presence. In marriage, communion allows two people from different backgrounds to bond emotionally, mentally, and spiritually.

"We proclaim to you what we have seen and heard, so that you also may have fellowship with us. And our fellowship is with the Father and with His Son, Jesus Christ." 1 John 1:3, NLT

Even as you're reading this book, we are fellowshipping—you and I are connecting over shared understanding. If that can happen through writing, how much more should communion happen in marriage, where partners are in close physical and emotional proximity?

Remember, communion is rooted in common union—common ground that joins two hearts together.

B. Common

The word common is not cheap or degrading. It means "to share the same interests, goals, and understanding with someone else."

"They continued steadfastly in… fellowship… Now all who believed were together, and had all things in common." Acts 2:42, 44, NKJV

The early believers shared so much in common that when grievances arose, they were free to express them. There was openness, not fear.

"Now in those days… a complaint arose against the Hebrews by the Hellenists, because their widows were neglected in the daily distribution." Acts 6:1, NKJV

Marriage is also a common union—a divine partnership between equals. God's original intent was that man and woman would become mates, irrespective of their background, culture, or age.

"Therefore a man shall leave his father and mother and be joined to his wife, and they shall become one flesh." Genesis 2:24, NKJV

The phrase **"both were naked and were not ashamed"** reflects the depth of bonding and transparency they shared. This is where compatibility is tested.

Compatibility and Shared Interests

Compatibility is "the ability to exist together without conflict" or "the ability to relate well with someone because of shared interests or values."

Ask yourself:

- What qualities attracted you to your spouse?
- How do you respond to your partner's views on sports, fashion, family, or career?
- Can you disagree respectfully and still find common ground?

Agreement doesn't always mean total conformity. Sometimes, it means agreeing to work through disagreements together.

"Can two people walk together unless they are agreed?" Amos 3:3, NKJV

When you entered marriage, you surrendered yourself to your spouse. That act of surrender created a sacred bond of fellowship. But when one spouse begins to pull away—emotionally, sexually, or spiritually—the union suffers. Saying "You can't have that; it's mine!" introduces division into what was meant to be one.

Only total surrender brings total communion, which produces love, understanding, and unity.

Final Thoughts

All human relationships—marital, social, political, or business —are sustained by communication based on common ground. Where no common interest exists, misunderstanding thrives. Where there is openness, agreement, and genuine connection, marriage flourishes.

2. Man's Involvement (Man's Position)

The institution of marriage was designed and established by God, as earlier scripturally and traditionally confirmed, but man was given the responsibility to consummate and steward it. Angelic beings and other spirit beings do not marry and therefore are not equipped to understand or participate in the dynamics of marriage. Marriage does not exist in heaven.

"They posed this question: 'Teacher, Moses gave us a law that if a man dies, leaving a wife but no children, his brother should marry the widow and have a child who will be the brother's heir... Finally, the woman died, too. So tell us, whose wife will she be in the resurrection? For all seven were married to her!' Jesus replied, 'Marriage is for people here on earth. But in the age to come, those worthy of being raised from the dead will neither marry nor be given in marriage.'" Luke 20:28–35, NLT

"For when they rise from the dead, they neither marry nor are given in marriage, but are like angels in heaven." Mark 12:25, NKJV

These scriptures make it clear: Marriage is an earthly ordinance, not a heavenly one. Angels were not created with marital features —no emotional needs, sexual organs, or flesh and blood. Paul affirmed this truth in his letter:

"What I am saying, dear brothers and sisters, is that flesh and blood cannot inherit the Kingdom of God." 1 Corinthians 15:50, NLT

This further affirms that marriage is carnal—designed for humanity in their earthly form. When God conceptualized marriage, He had man in mind. Genesis 2:18 reflects this:

"And the Lord God said, 'It is not good that the man should be alone; I will make him a helper comparable to him.'"

What is Marriage?

There are various definitions of marriage. The Merriam-Webster

Dictionary defines it as:

"The state of being united to a person of the opposite sex as husband or wife in a consensual and contractual relationship recognized by law."

The Longman Dictionary of Contemporary English says: "A legal agreement between a man and a woman to bond them together into one."

But here's a more practical and biblical understanding:

"Marriage is a mutual agreement and understanding between a man and a woman who choose to unite and live as one, with the purpose of complementing and supporting each other."

In summary, marriage is a lifelong contract between two consenting adults of the opposite sex, regardless of their family, race, or creed. It is a covenant built on commitment, unity, and purpose

Marriage Is Carnal

The topic of "Marriage is Carnal" will likely generate many questions, criticisms, and strong reactions—especially from religious minds who may be unwilling to hear perspectives that challenge their spiritual assumptions. Yet, many Christian couples struggle in marriage precisely because they have over-spiritualized the institution.

From the beginning, marriage was not spiritual in form. God Himself designed marriage for mankind while on earth—not in heaven or in the spirit realm. Let's revisit the foundational passage:

"And the Lord God said, 'It is not good that the man should be alone; I will make him a helper comparable to him.'… But for Adam there was not found a helper comparable to him. And the Lord God caused a deep sleep to fall on Adam, and he slept; and He took one of his ribs, and closed up the flesh in its place. Then the rib which the Lord God had taken from man He made into a woman, and He brought her to the man. And Adam said: 'This is now bone of my bones and flesh of my flesh; she shall be called Woman, because she was taken out of Man.'" Genesis 2:18, 20–23, NKJV

This act was not spiritual in nature but physical and emotional. God recognized a human need and provided a human solution—companionship and partnership in the flesh.

i.   Paul's Perspective on Earthly Responsibility

Apostle Paul echoed this reality when he wrote to the Corinthian church:

"I want you to be without care. He who is unmarried cares for the things of the Lord—how he may please the Lord. But he who is married cares about the things of the world—how he may please his wife. There is a difference between a wife and a virgin. The unmarried woman cares about the things of the Lord... But she who is married cares about the things of the world—how she may please her husband." 1 Corinthians 7:32–34, NLT

Here, Paul clearly shows that marriage introduces divided attention, as the married person must now be concerned with earthly responsibilities. This is not a condemnation of marriage—it is simply the truth that marriage is carnal, in the sense that it involves the physical, emotional, and practical realities of life.

ii.   Spirituality Must Not Override Marital Responsibility

The rise of hyper-spiritual attitudes toward marriage has done great harm in many Christian homes. Some believers wrongly assume that spiritual pursuits should override marital obligations—but the Bible warns against this imbalance.

"Do not deprive one another except with consent for a time that you may give yourselves to fasting and prayer; and come together again so that Satan does not tempt you because of your lack of self-control." 1 Corinthians 7:5, NKJV

This passage clearly commands spouses not to withhold intimacy, except temporarily and only with mutual agreement. God does not approve of using spirituality as an excuse to deny marital duty.

A True-Life Example

There was once a Christian couple—both fervent believers—who fell into this trap. Though married, they neither bathed together nor engaged in intimacy. While they shared the same bed, they turned their backs on each other, driven by a flawed understanding of holiness.

Years passed, and they grew anxious over their inability to conceive. Seeking divine intervention, they went to their pastor for counseling. During the session, it was revealed they had never consummated their marriage. When asked why, they quoted Scripture out of context:

"The body is not for sexual immorality but for the Lord and the Lord for the body… Do you not know that your bodies are temples of the Holy Spirit…?" 1 Corinthians 6:13–20, NKJV

This is a misapplication of Scripture. These verses were never meant to suggest that sex within marriage is unholy. In fact, sexual intimacy between husband and wife is God-ordained.

"And Adam knew (had sexual relations with) Eve his wife, and she conceived and bore Cain…" Genesis 4:1, NKJV

God's original design includes physical union as a vital part of marital fulfillment. The Bible even affirms that:

"And they were both naked, the man and his wife, and were not ashamed." Genesis 2:25, NKJV

This was literal, not symbolic. There was complete openness, physical vulnerability, and acceptance between husband and wife. You are to cover your nakedness from everyone—except your spouse.

> iii.   Marriage Requires Physical Expression

Whether you were once deeply spiritual as a single person, the moment thoughts of marriage begin to enter your heart, a shift occurs. Physical and emotional dimensions must now be embraced. You begin to think not only about pleasing the Lord but also about pleasing your spouse.

Marriage introduces divided devotion—but this is not sinful; it is by divine design.

iv.   Balance Is Key

The irony is that you cannot sacrifice your spouse on the altar of spirituality, nor should you forsake God for your marriage. Both are necessary. A balanced life will keep you fruitful spiritually and fulfilled maritally.

- Serve God with your heart and soul.

- Love your spouse with your body and affection.

- Do not allow spiritual pride to make you fail in your primary assignment at home.

Final Thought

Marriage is carnal—not sinful—but physical, emotional, and practical. God created it that way. Spirituality enhances marriage but should never replace your God-given responsibility to your spouse. A successful marriage requires a spiritual foundation, yes—but it must also be built with the bricks of emotional connection, physical intimacy, and mutual care.

"The two shall become one flesh." Genesis 2:24

Let no one—especially not your misapplied spirituality—separate what God has joined together.

3. Seduction in Marriage – Is It Necessary?

The word seduction is often misunderstood in the context of marriage. Typically defined as "the act of enticing or attracting someone to sexual intimacy, especially in a way that is charming, appealing, or irresistible," seduction—within the bounds of marriage—is not only appropriate, but essential. It is a vital ingredient in sustaining emotional and sexual intimacy between husband and wife.

Some may ask, "Why must I seduce my spouse? After all, I already have legal and spiritual access to them whenever I desire." This attitude is common but dangerously shortsighted. Many married individuals forget that marriage becomes what you make of it. If left neglected, it grows stale. If nurtured, it flourishes.

Before marriage, most men go to great lengths to win a woman's affection—sending romantic texts, buying thoughtful gifts, planning special dates, and showing constant admiration. Many women also invest emotionally and physically, preparing themselves to attract and captivate. However, once the vows are exchanged and the honeymoon fades, these efforts often fade too.

God Designed Sex to Be Enjoyed in Marriage

The Life Application Bible commentary on 1 Corinthians 6:18 says, "God created sex to be a beautiful and essential ingredient of marriage." The fulfillment of sexual desire is not a one-sided obligation—it is mutual. And just like a good meal, intimacy must be thoughtfully prepared—not rushed or taken for granted. If the sexual appeal in a marriage is not guarded and continually refreshed, it may lose its flavor.

"Salt is good for seasoning. But if it loses its flavor, how do you make it salty again? Flavorless salt is good neither for the soil nor for fertilizer. It is thrown away. Anyone who is willing to hear should listen and understand!" Luke 14:34–35, NLT

This is why many marriages fall victim to external seductions. When the bedroom becomes boring and uninviting, the natural craving for excitement and attention may lead a spouse to look elsewhere. But when you consistently repackage the same love and attraction in new and meaningful ways, your spouse will always be drawn back to you—like a hungry lion returning to fresh prey.

Have you ever wondered?

a "Why is my husband enticed by every woman in a skirt?"

b. "Why does my wife seem emotionally drawn to other men?"

The answer may lie not in what those outsiders possess, but in how they present themselves. Seduction is a skill. Whether consciously or not others are actively competing for your spouse's attention. Ignoring this reality leaves your marriage vulnerable to temptation.

"Woe to the world because of offenses! For offenses (temptations) must come..." Matthew 18:7, NKJV

When a spouse is denied satisfaction or neglected emotionally or sexually, the resulting craving can become difficult to suppress. This is how temptation takes root.

"And remember, when you are being tempted, do not say, 'God is tempting me.' God is never tempted to do wrong, and He never tempts anyone else. Temptation comes from our own desires, which entice us and drag us away. These desires give birth to sinful actions..." James 1:13–15, NLT

So while this chapter is not strictly about temptation, understanding it helps us appreciate why seduction within marriage is a spiritual and emotional necessity.

4. Understanding Your Partner

A key factor in marital conflict is the failure to understand the differences between men and women. These differences —biological, emotional, and psychological—were intentionally designed by God. Attempting to blur or exchange these roles causes dysfunction and frustration.

"He took one of Adam's ribs and closed up the place from which He had taken it. Then the Lord God made a woman from the rib." Genesis 2:21–22, NLT

Though woman came from man, she was uniquely fashioned. Hormonal differences between the sexes account for many of their distinctions—how they think, feel, respond, and express love. This is why men are typically more rational, and women more emotional. He may want it logical; she wants it poetic. She cries; he ponders.

These differences do not mean one is weaker than the other. In fact, the notion of women being "weaker vessels" has often been misinterpreted. Women endure physical and emotional cycles that many men could not handle. Childbirth alone testifies to their strength.

"Husbands… dwell with them with understanding, giving honor to the wife, as to the weaker vessel…" 1 Peter 3:7, NKJV

This refers to emotional sensitivity, not inferiority. Understanding these differences will help both spouses appreciate one another more deeply. Neither is complete without the other. When a husband learns to honor his wife's emotions, and a wife respects her husband's logic, unity is strengthened.

5. Sexual Needs Are Different—But Equally Important

Hormonal and emotional differences affect sexual desires as well. Dr. Gary and Barbara Rosberg, in their book "Five Love Needs of Men and Women", stress the importance of meeting each other's needs. They write:

"You need to know your spouse's heart and needs, and then sacrificially step away from your own selfishness and learn—really learn—how to meet those needs... When you meet the needs of your spouse, you are fulfilling your marriage vows."

They warn that neglecting your spouse's needs can cost you your marriage. Many couples enter into a silent contract of "fifty-fifty performance"—offering affection only when it's returned. But love is not a trade. It's a sacrifice. And seduction is a part of that sacrifice.

"When our love needs go unmet... the results are not pretty. Perhaps the bottom-line reason for meeting your spouse's needs is that if you don't, you could end up losing him or her to another."

Final Thoughts:

Seduction Is Sacred in Marriage

To seduce your spouse is not sinful—it is godly. It is part of the beautiful dance of love God intended to exist in marriage. It rekindles passion. It keeps temptation at bay. It reminds your spouse that they are desirable, wanted, and cherished.

Do not let your marriage lose its flavor. Continually season it with affection, admiration, and seduction. Keep the fires of intimacy burning, not just in body but in soul.

"Let your fountain be blessed, and rejoice with the wife of your youth... be enraptured always with her love." Proverbs 5:18–19, NKJV

6. Top Five Love Needs of Husbands and Wives

A comprehensive survey conducted among over 700 couples revealed the distinct love needs of men and women. The findings highlight how emotional and physical intimacy are prioritized differently between the sexes:

Husbands' Top Five Love Need	Wives' Top Five Love Needs:
1. Unconditional Love & Acceptance	1. Unconditional Love & Acceptance
2. Sexual Intimacy	2. Emotional Intimacy & Communication
3 .Companionship	3. Spiritual Intimacy
4. Encouragement & Affirmation	4. Encouragement & Affirmation
5. Spiritual Intimacy	5. Companionship

It is clear from the chart that sexual intimacy ranks second for men, while for women, emotional intimacy and communication hold that position. This difference is significant: what a man often views as a core need, a woman may view as a result of emotional closeness.

A man often connects through physical touch and sexual expression. A woman, however, is more likely to crave conversation, affection, and emotional presence. Understanding this difference is not to create division but to help couples intentionally meet each other's needs in love.

As Dr. Gary Rosberg notes, "Meeting your spouse's love needs is not optional—it is the very heart of the marriage covenant."

7. Understanding the Cleaving Concept

"Therefore a man shall leave his father and mother and be joined to his wife, and they shall become one flesh." Genesis 2:24, NKJV

At the heart of marital success is the cleaving concept—a principle so critical that it was emphasized both in the Old Testament (Genesis 2:24) and reaffirmed by Jesus in the New Testament (Matthew 19:5).

The Hebrew word translated "cleave" is "dābāq", which means "to cling to, stick to, or glue to." The Greek equivalent in Matthew 19:5 is "proskollaō", also meaning "to glue together." These are not passive actions. They are intentional commitments to emotional, physical, and spiritual unity.

Cleaving Requires Leaving

To cleave, one must first leave—not with bitterness or disrespect— but with maturity. Leaving doesn't mean cutting off your family; it means redefining priorities and boundaries.

Marriage creates a new family unit. Until a man or woman detaches emotionally and mentally from their family of origin, they will struggle to fully bond with their spouse.

"Therefore, a man shall leave (detach from) his father and mother (family of origin) and cleave (stick, unite) to his wife, and they shall become one flesh." Genesis 2:24, emphasis mine

In many African cultures, especially in Nigeria, this principle is challenged by the deep integration of extended family systems. This has given rise to terms like "our wife" instead of "my wife." However, Scripture clearly emphasizes individual responsibility and unity within marriage.

The inability of couples to emotionally and mentally detach from their parents and siblings often leads to interference, confusion, and broken communication. No matter how close you are to your family, once married, your primary loyalty shifts to your spouse.

The Psychological Bond of Family

There's no denying the deep emotional connection children have with their parents and siblings. It is within that environment they formed their first understanding of love, safety, and trust.

"Can a woman forget her nursing child, and not have compassion on the son of her womb?" Isaiah 49:15, NKJV

"Reuben was secretly planning to help Joseph escape… Judah said, 'What can we gain by killing our brother? That would just give us a guilty conscience.'" Genesis 37:21–22, 26, NLT

These scriptures reflect how strong emotional ties run in family lines. But in marriage, those ties must be resituated, not erased, so the new union can be nourished without conflict or division.

Marriage Must Be Nurtured

Marriage is like a new organization or an infant plant—it needs nurturing, understanding, and protection. Without proper boundaries, even loving families can become unintentional intruders in your union.

Marital bliss is elusive for many because they never fully embrace the cleaving principle. They live under the influence of extended family expectations and fail to form a true partnership with their spouse.

God's plan was not to dissolve the extended family but to establish priority in intimacy. You can respect your parents and siblings, but your first commitment must now be to your spouse. The inability to do this leads to isolation, suspicion, and emotional detachment between couples.

Quoting Dr. Norman Vincent Peale on Cleaving

Dr. Peale rightly captured the essence of biblical oneness in his commentary on Matthew 19:4–6:

"A man by himself may have strength and determination and aggressiveness, but he's not complete. A woman may have great sensitivity and intuition and feminine insight, but she's not complete either. These incomplete units are designed to become one unit, to fit together like pieces of a jigsaw puzzle… Marriage is a fusion of two opposite beings in harmony with divine law."

This fusion is not just physical—it is emotional, mental, spiritual, and practical. The man brings his strength, vision, and discipline; the woman brings her compassion, discernment, and nurturing spirit. Together, they form a powerful whole, a covenant bond that no outsider has the right to interfere with.

"What God has joined together let no man put asunder." Matthew 19:6, NKJV

Cleaving Builds Covenant Intimacy

Marriage is not about cohabiting under the same roof. It's about joining your hearts, your minds, and your lives. It's about leaving, cleaving, and building a new foundation together. It's about seeing your spouse not as "a part of the family," but as "your family."

Until cleaving happens, real intimacy cannot be birthed.

Let your marriage reflect this divine principle—detach with love, cleave with purpose, and grow in covenant intimacy.

Rejuvenating Marital Bliss

Marriage is a divine institution, designed by God and entrusted to man for consummation. While the framework was divinely inspired, its success hinges on man's active participation, guided by scriptural principles and practical wisdom. When one partner begins to ignore the other—emotionally, physically, or spiritually—the harmony of the union begins to erode.

Bitterness takes root. Words, once loving, begin to cut. Resentment morphs into anger and jealousy. If unchecked, this can spiral into separation, divorce, and emotional estrangement. Yet, even the deepest rift can be healed—if detected early and addressed with humility and intentionality.

What many marriages need is not a dramatic overhaul, but a simple renewal of the vow to love, honor, and cherish. This chapter offers practical insights that help fan the ember of love back into flame, strengthening the bond between spouses.

The Appreciation Concept

* ❖ When was the last time you gave your spouse a gift outside special occasions like birthdays, anniversaries, or Valentine's Day?

And if you did, was it just to appease, impress, or manipulate forgiveness—or was it purely to say "I appreciate you"?

When last did you compliment your spouse for:

* ❖ A new hairstyle?
* ❖ Their dressing or fragrance?
* ❖ How well they manage the home or care for the children?
* ❖ Their role as a husband or wife, or even their contribution to your sexual satisfaction?

Too often, couples take for granted the very things that should be celebrated. Yet, appreciation is the water that helps love grow. It tells your partner, "I see you," "You matter to me," and "I don't take you for granted."

Even simple words like:

    a. "I love you"

    b. "You're the best thing that's ever happened to me"

    c. "What would life be without you?"

… Spoken outside the bedroom, rekindle connection and intimacy.

Dating Shouldn't End After the Wedding

Many couples abandon dating after they marry, thinking it's only for courtship. This is a grave mistake.

Dating your spouse is one of the healthiest habits you can maintain. It's not about luxury or splurging—it's about intentional time spent together.

1. Go on walks.

2. Have lunch at a quiet spot.

3. Steal away for evening conversations.

4. Surprise them with flowers or favorite snacks.

5. Recreate your first date.

These simple acts work wonders in reviving affection and deepening emotional intimacy. As long as you want to enjoy the best of your marriage—even into old age—you must continue to invest in it.

The Power of Daily Connection

Marriage thrives on communication. Make it a point to connect outside of bedtime routines. My wife and I, for example, have what we call "Our Gossip Time"—a moment set aside to talk about our day, laugh, share thoughts, and simply be together. These moments have become precious to us, helping us stay emotionally aligned.

You don't need long hours. Even ten undistracted minutes a day can change the atmosphere in your marriage.

The Ministry of Reassurance

One of the deepest needs in marriage is the need to feel safe in love —to know that, in this person, I have a home.

"Place me like a seal over your heart, like a seal on your arm; for love is as strong as death… It burns like blazing fire, like a mighty flame. Many waters cannot quench love." Song of Songs 8:6–7, NIV

When your spouse is secure in your love, they will not seek affirmation or fulfillment elsewhere. Reassurance is a ministry of consistency—you say "I love you", but more importantly, you prove it daily through your actions, words, and presence.

Love is like a rose. It may start strong, but it needs watering—not once a year, but consistently. It must be fed with kindness, praise, attention, and forgiveness.

Marriage: A Lifelong School

Mrs. Betty Irabor, publisher of Genevieve Magazine, once said in an interview with The Punch newspaper:

"Marriage is a relationship where you continue to learn, sometimes with long-suffering. Sometimes you learn to be the humble party to say, 'You are wrong.' You learn not to take each other for granted. Marriage is the only institution that issues you a certificate before you ever start—therefore, you never graduate from it until death."

Marriage is the only institution that gives you a certificate on Day One. Every other institution requires training before certification, but not marriage. That alone should humble us to keep learning, growing, and nurturing.

Final Thoughts

Marital bliss is not reserved for a chosen few. It is attainable by those willing to work, love, and grow. The process is not mystical

—it is practical:

Learn to say "Thank you" and "I'm sorry."

- ➤ Never stop dating your spouse.
- ➤ Share quality time.
- ➤ Appreciate the little things.
- ➤ Reassure your partner of your love.
- ➤ Stay teachable.

You cannot stop working on your marriage and expect it to flourish. Like a garden, it thrives where it is watered. And when both partners surrender in love to each other under God, they will not only survive, but thrive—joyfully, fruitfully, and passionately.

Contemporary View of Marriage (Worldview)

Like many other God-ordained institutions, the institution of marriage has undergone significant modifications over the centuries. While originally rooted in divine intent, it has been reshaped—positively or negatively—by societal ideologies and cultural evolution. Across the world today, the concept of marriage varies greatly. What is accepted in the West might not be acceptable in the Orient, among Arabs, or in African traditional society.

Historically, monogamy—defined as the custom of being married to one person at a time—was the foundational marital structure. However, over time, civilization introduced alternatives such as polygamy, bigamy, and same-sex marriages, creating moral and ideological tension between scriptural values and societal trends.

Polygamy in Historical Perspective

In her book Christian Marriage in Africa, Adrian Hastings (Chapter 2, pp. 29–30) highlights a compelling comparison of marriage traditions across continents. She notes that many of the practices seen in ancient Israel and early European societies, such as bride-price and even wife purchase, have strong parallels in African traditions. For instance: "The bride-wealth of Africa is paralleled by the 'weotuma' or wife purchase of ancient English society, which continued long after they had become Christians… if polygamy was never a widespread part of the marriage system of the West—as it was in Asia—a great deal of successive polygamy… did exist."

Her point is clear: Marriage customs are not static, nor are they exclusive to certain cultures. And while modern "Western marriage" often emphasizes individual choice, romantic love, and the nuclear family, historical evidence shows a blend of practices —many of which today would be classified as non-monogamous or polygamous.

The Origin of Polygamy

Polygamy, especially as first recorded in Scripture, finds its origin in Lamech, the fifth-generation descendant of Cain:

"Lamech married two women—Adah and Zillah." Genesis 4:19, NLT

This act marked a clear departure from God's original plan of monogamy. Lamech's polygamous choice wasn't driven by divine instruction, but seemingly by lust, rebellion, and pride. His bold declaration in Genesis 4:23–24 reveals a defiant spirit—one that mocks both divine order and accountability.

Polygamy, in this sense, represents man's deliberate distortion of God's design, driven by selfish cravings and unwillingness to be governed by moral constraints.

"Have you eaten the fruit I commanded you not to eat?" "Yes," Adam admitted, "but it was the woman You gave me who brought me the fruit, and I ate it." Genesis 3:11–12, NLT

From the Garden of Eden, man began to shift blame, rationalize disobedience, and eventually shape institutions like marriage in his own image. This ushered in not only polygamy, but a wide range of deviations from God's perfect design.

Humanism and the Redefinition of Marriage

In Hope for America's Last Generation (p. 119), Galyn Wiemers quotes the Humanist Society of Western New York, formed by John Dewey:

"Humanism is a joyous alternative to religions that believe in a supernatural God and life in the hereafter... People are best able to solve the world's problems when free to think for themselves, using reason and knowledge as their tools."

This modern worldview—humanism—denies divine authority and promotes self-governance. It is this same worldview that fuels redefinitions of marriage to suit man's ideological conveniences, including polygamy, same-sex unions, and open relationships.

Polygamy: Merits and Demerits

While Scripture and Christian doctrine uphold monogamy, it is also important to understand the arguments often made for polygamy, especially within cultural and historical contexts.

Merits of Polygamy (Cultural Justifications)

1. Procreation and Posterity: In traditional societies, the production of many children was vital for the survival of clans and tribes. Polygamy was a strategy to combat childlessness or secure male offspring (see Judges 8:30).

2. Economic or Political Alliance: Marriages were often used to forge ties between powerful families or tribes (1 Kings 3:1–2).

3. Sexual Cravings: Some pursued polygamy simply to satisfy insatiable sexual desires (2 Chronicles 11:23).

4. Workforce Expansion: In agrarian economies, large families meant more hands to work on farms (Genesis 16:1,3).

5. Social Protection for Women: In societies with gender imbalances, polygamy offered marriage and protection to otherwise vulnerable women.

Demerits of Polygamy

a) It promotes jealousy, rivalry, and emotional neglect among wives.

b) It often undermines intimacy between husband and wife.

c) It distracts from the "one flesh" concept instituted by God (Genesis 2:24).

d) It can become a tool for objectifying women, reducing marriage to utility and procreation alone.

e) It frequently stems from lust and ego, rather than love and covenant.

Polygamy in the Old Testament

The Old Testament does not give a direct condemnation of polygamy. Patriarchs like Jacob, David, and Solomon practiced it—often with dire consequences. Although Mosaic Law emphasized moral and social order, it neither promoted nor strictly prohibited polygamy. Instead, laws such as the Levirate marriage (Genesis 38:8, Deuteronomy 25:5–10) indirectly permitted multiple marriages for lineage preservation.

However, the New Testament brings clarity to God's ideal. Jesus, in Matthew 19:4–6, reaffirms the Genesis standard:

"From the beginning, God made them male and female... the two shall become one flesh. Therefore, what God has joined together, let no one separate."

Paul echoes the same principle in 1 Timothy 3:2, instructing that a church leader must be "the husband of one wife."

Islamic Perspective on Polygamy

In Islam, polygamy (up to four wives) is permitted under specific regulations, often viewed as a form of social justice, allowing men to assist families burdened by poverty or surplus female children. However, Islamic law also insists on equal treatment of all wives, a condition many fail to uphold in practice.

Conclusion

Polygamy, while historically widespread and culturally rationalized, remains a deviation from God's original design. Its roots are tied more to human indulgence and societal constructs than divine will.

As believers, we are not called to conform to the world's shifting ideologies but to uphold biblical principles of love, fidelity, and covenant. As Paul admonishes in Romans 12:2:

"Do not be conformed to this world, but be transformed by the renewing of your mind..."

Marriage is not merely a contract or cultural norm—it is a spiritual covenant, a reflection of Christ's love for His Church. Let us return to that sacred blueprint.

Polygamy — Its De-Merits and Contemporary Relevance

Understanding the Cost of Polygamy

The de-merits of polygamy are better imagined than experienced. Many Africans—whether on the maternal or paternal side—have experienced the realities of polygamous homes. This form of marriage is particularly prevalent in African societies due to a combination of factors:

- ❖ Limited access to education and global exposure

- ❖ The extended family system

- ❖ Deep-rooted communal values that override the nuclear family unit

These traditional structures have nurtured a culture where polygamy thrives, often normalized under social, economic, or cultural justifications.

Approved and Unapproved Polygamy

There are generally two forms of polygamy observed in practice:

1. Approved Polygamy: The polygamist houses all wives together

under one roof, maintaining a visible and unified family system.

2. Unapproved Polygamy: The man resides with one wife while secretly maintaining apartments elsewhere for other wives or concubines. This is especially common in urbanized areas.

Because marriage is often seen more as a communal project than a personal covenant, partner selection is sometimes dictated by family elders, bypassing the couple's emotional compatibility. In some cases, widows of deceased male relatives are inherited by next-of-kin; further perpetuating polygamy and its complications.

The Chaos Within: Polygamy in Practice

It is a fallacy to advocate for an "ideal" polygamous family. In reality, polygamous homes are almost always plagued by:

- Jealousy and rivalry among wives

- Sibling competition and conflict

- Emotional manipulation and schemes to outwit one another

Imagine the effort it takes to build a healthy relationship with one spouse—then multiply that by two or more. Emotional fairness becomes impossible.

"Solomon had seven hundred wives and three hundred concubines. And sure enough, they led his heart away from the Lord..." 1 Kings 11:3–4, NLT

"No one can serve two masters. For you will hate one and love the other..." Matthew 6:24, NLT

It is easier for ten men to share a room than for two women to peacefully share a home, regardless of their status.

Even among sisters, rivalry flared between Rachel and Leah, as recorded in Genesis 30:1–16. Their interactions depict resentment, jealousy, bargaining over intimacy, and emotional manipulation. Polygamy breeds such emotional chaos.

Consequences on Children and Society

Polygamy doesn't only affect wives—it deeply scars the children. Mothers, driven by insecurity and competition, often sow seeds of division, rivalry, and manipulation among their children.

"Just do what I tell you. Go out and get the goats…" — Genesis 27:6–13, NLT

Such manipulative parenting leads to broken relationships, greed, corruption, and a society shaped by individuals conditioned to survive through schemes rather than truth

A Personal Witness Against Polygamy

The author of this book writes from firsthand experience. Raised in a polygamous home, I can boldly say: "It was a form of hell I would not wish even on my enemy."

At the age of 8 or 9, during a casual chat with my father, I told him: "Papa, I will never marry more than one wife in my life, no matter what happens."

My father was shocked. He asked:

1. "What if your wife is barren?"

I answered, "I'd rather live with her without children than marry another."

2. "What if she cheats or tries to poison you?"

My response: "I will forgive her and continue with her."

By the grace of God, I have kept that vow. I married my one and only wife on December 28, 1991, and we are still together.

Polygamy Is No Longer Justifiable

In today's world of exposure, scientific advancement, and scriptural clarity, polygamy is not a solution but a problem.

- Childlessness: Adoption or IVF are viable alternatives.

- Infidelity: Forgiveness and counseling are better responses than replacement.

"Most important of all, continue to show deep love for each other, for love covers a multitude of sins." 1 Peter 4:8, NLT

"Disregarding another person's faults preserves love…" Proverbs 17:9, NLT

"Get rid of all bitterness, rage, anger… forgiving one another, just as God through Christ has forgiven you." Ephesians 4:31–32, NLT

Polygamy may have been tolerated in ignorance, but in light of Scripture and reason, it cannot be defended today.

Islamic Perspective on Polygamy

In Islam, marriage is both a religious duty and moral safeguard. It provides an outlet for sexual needs and a basis for societal structure. Islam teaches monogamy but permits polygamy (up to four wives) under strict conditions—chiefly fair treatment and justice among the wives.

"In a way you can treat your wives justly, even though you may wish to do that…" Qur'an, Surah 4:129

"Prophet, we have made lawful to you the wives… and any believing woman who gives herself to you…" Surah 33:50

To a devout Muslim, polygamy is seen as an obligation, not a choice to be taken lightly. But this theory has practical challenges. Can a man love and treat all wives equally? Can he meet all their emotional and physical needs without preference?

"Elkanah had two wives… he loved Hannah very much… but her adversary provoked her sore…" 1 Samuel 1:2–6, NLT

Even when intentioned with fairness, grudges, favoritism, and emotional neglect creep in. Polygamy, though culturally or religiously permitted, often becomes a breeding ground for heartache, inequality, and broken trust.

"No one can serve two masters…" Matthew 6:24, NLT

Conclusion

Polygamy may have historic and cultural roots, but it cannot be justified in light of love, grace, and biblical truth. Marriage, as God ordained, is between one man and one woman, bonded in love and mutual submission.

"Therefore, a man shall leave his father and mother and be joined to his wife, and they shall become one flesh." Genesis 2:24

Let us choose the biblical model of marriage, where love is undivided, forgiveness is constant, and unity is preserved.

Blueprint for Marriage

Understanding Monogamy

Monogamy is the divinely instituted system of marriage involving one man and one woman, committed exclusively to one another for life. It is a covenantal relationship that excludes any third party, reflecting God's original intent at the dawn of creation.

"Therefore a man shall leave his father and mother and be joined to his wife, and they shall become one flesh. And they were both naked, the man and his wife, and were not ashamed." Genesis 2:24–25, NKJV

This biblical model of monogamous union has stood as the foundation of marriage throughout history until recent times, when evolving ideologies like same-sex marriage, polyandry, and humanistic philosophies began to challenge God's divine order.-

The Rise of Humanism and the Attack on Divine Order

As mentioned earlier, humanism is the belief that man possesses within himself all he needs for life and happiness, without reference to a higher being. This ideology rejects God's sovereignty and exalts human reason above divine truth. As a result, family values and moral foundations have come under intense attack in today's society.

Same-sex marriage, for example, is a product of such reasoning —a clear deviation from the divine pattern. In countries like Nigeria, such unions remain proscribed due to moral, religious, and cultural convictions rooted in traditional and scriptural principles.

Jesus' Affirmation of Monogamy

When questioned about divorce, Jesus Christ didn't just talk about separation—He affirmed God's original pattern for marriage:

"Haven't you read the Scriptures?" Jesus replied. "They record that from the beginning 'God made them male and female.' And He said, 'This explains why a man leaves his father and mother and is joined to his wife, and the two are united into one.' Since they are no longer two but one, let no one split apart what God has joined together." Matthew 19:4–6, NLT

Here, Jesus refers to one man, one woman—not multiple spouses or same-gender unions. This truth forms the bedrock of Christian marriage and the identity of the Christian family.

Apostolic Teaching on Monogamy

The Apostles Paul and Peter also upheld monogamy as the only acceptable form of Christian marriage. For leaders in the church, marital purity was a qualification:

"A bishop then must be blameless, the husband of one wife..." 1 Timothy 3:2, NKJV

> "Likewise deacons must be the husbands of one wife, ruling their children and their own houses well." 1 Timothy 3:12, NKJV

Even though polygamy was tolerated under the Mosaic law, especially during the Old Testament era and among post-exilic Jews, the Christian ideal has always been monogamous marriage —a covenant between one man and one woman under God.

The Beauty and Merits of Monogamy

Monogamy provides a stable platform for intimacy, commitment, and personal growth within marriage. It enables couples to:

a. Explore their individual personalities in depth

b. Build trust, loyalty, and understanding over time

c. Raise children in a stable, loving environment

d. Strengthen the emotional and spiritual bond between husband and wife

Marriage is a lifelong commitment, requiring daily work and intentional investment. Mrs. Ruth Stafford Peale, in her book "Secrets of Staying in Love" (pg. 10), described marriage beautifully:

"Marriage as a lifelong contract is so exciting and potentially rewarding—living with someone, studying them, supporting them, liberating their strengths, compensating for their weaknesses, and helping them soar as they were designed to."

Marriage is a relationship of three: God, the man, and the woman. This divine triangle ensures the couple remains grounded and guided.

Common Sense and Scriptural Clarity

It takes common sense and spiritual insight to discern that God never intended marriage to be polygamous or same-sex. If polygamy were His plan, He could have taken many ribs from Adam to create multiple women—but instead, He took only one rib and formed one woman.

"And the LORD God said, 'It is not good that man should be alone; I will make him a helper comparable to him.' ... And the rib which the Lord God had taken from man, He made into a woman, and He brought her to the man." Genesis 2:18, 21–22, NKJV

"At last!" the man exclaimed. "This one is bone from my bone, and flesh from my flesh!" Genesis 2:23, NLT

There's no room in the creation account for multiple wives or same-sex unions. The divine blueprint is clear—one man and one woman, united in love and purpose.

The Spiritual Responsibility of Monogamy

Monogamy demands that we study our spouse—learn their strengths, understand their weaknesses, appreciate their uniqueness, and commit to building a life together.

"Let the husband render to his wife the affection due her, and likewise also the wife to her husband." 1 Corinthians 7:3, NKJV

"Study your spouse as though they were a rare, fascinating creation. Learn their moods, values, likes, and dislikes." Mrs. Ruth Stafford Peale

This lifelong study leads to a deep emotional and spiritual connection that polygamy cannot offer. It is in this process of learning and loving one person deeply that marriage becomes a sacred adventure.

A Final Word

Polygamy and same-sex marriages are not only cultural deviations—they are spiritual rebellions against God's established order. The world may present arguments for these systems, but Scripture remains firm and unchanging:

"He who made them at the beginning 'made them male and female.'" Matthew 19:4, NKJV

"He created them male and female and blessed them..." Genesis 5:1–2, NKJV

Any deviation from this divine structure reflects man's failure to submit to God's design. As believers, we are called not to conform to the world's standards but to live by God's original intent.

Let us champion monogamy, not just as a biblical ideal but as a practical pathway to healthy, joyful, and lasting marriages

CHAPTER 2:

Cultural Perspectives on Marriage

Culture is defined as "the beliefs, way of life, art, and customs that are shared and accepted by people in a particular society." Seventy to eighty percent of who we are stems from our culture, making it a major influence in our socio-economic lifestyles. Every individual is a product of a particular culture, and our behaviors and mannerisms often reflect this reality.

Due to these cultural differences, integration among people of diverse backgrounds—race, tribe, or tongue—can be difficult. Whether you are religious or non-religious, your thoughts, beliefs, and upbringing influence your relationship and marriage. Cultural practices come with their own set of rules, guidelines, and values—some positive, others not so.

While some cultural traditions are not inherently negative, they can shape perspectives on finances, parenting, communication, and even gender roles. When partners from different cultures come together in marriage, differences often surface. These can either become opportunities for growth or sources of conflict.

Culture's Influence on Marriage

Marriage is the most intimate and important relationship between a man and a woman. It involves integrating two worlds —cultures, values, and habits—into one. These differences may not be obvious at the start of a relationship but often emerge over time. As history tells us, humanity once shared a common language and culture until God intervened at Babel.

"At one time the whole world spoke a single language... That is why the city was called Babel, because it was there that the Lord confused the people by giving them many languages, thus scattering them across the earth." Genesis 11:1-9 NLT

Culture influences everything from choosing a spouse to the wedding ceremony, bride-price, and family expectations. Some cultural heritages impose restrictions based on tribe, language, status, and religious background. Inter-tribal or inter-cultural marriages were once forbidden, as seen in the Bible:

"Do not intermarry with them... They will lead your young people away from Me to worship other gods." Deuteronomy 7:2–4 NLT

However, the world has since become a global village. People from different tribes and nations have fused in many ways. Some language and cultural barriers are fading, making it easier to connect across borders.

"Ruth fell at his feet and thanked him warmly. 'Why are you being so kind to me?' she asked. 'I am only a foreigner. Yes, I know," Boaz replied. "But I also know about the love and kindness you have shown..." Ruth 2:10–11 NLT

Couples must acknowledge cultural differences, communicate openly, and address expectations. Marital success lies in being sensitive to each other's backgrounds without compromising Biblical standards. As Christian philosopher Gideon Strauss once said: "There is clearly a need for the courageous and innovative use of cultural elements that do not stand in contradiction to Biblical truth, while avoiding the temptation of compromising authentic Christian faith."

Cultural Conflict in Marriage

In culturally conservative families, men may be overly dominant, suppressing mutual respect and affection. A woman from a background where yelling or hitting is normalized may carry these behaviors into her marriage—until she unlearns them. Cultural practices should never replace love, kindness, and Biblical values.

"Submit to one another out of reverence for Christ." Ephesians 5:21 NLT

"Wives, submit to your husbands as you do to the Lord. For a husband is the head of his wife as Christ is the head of the church." Ephesians 5:22–23 NLT

It's important to uphold the sanctity of marriage over culture. Your spouse is more important than your heritage.

The Role of In-Laws

In-laws play a vital role in a married couple's life. Balancing your own needs with that of a new family isn't easy, but it's worth the effort. Healthy boundaries, respect, and clear communication are essential.

Key Tips for Navigating In-Laws:

- Work with Your Spouse: Don't force them to choose between you and their family. You're a team.

- Set Boundaries: Decide as a couple what's acceptable. Don't overextend yourself.

- Communicate Directly: Avoid relaying messages through your spouse.

- Know Yourself: Don't change who you are to please others.

- Be Realistic: Not all in-laws fit stereotypes—some are kind, others difficult.

- Stay Mature: Learn to navigate differences with grace.

- Be Kind: If you can't say anything nice, stay silent and smile.

- Don't Undermine: Always respect your spouse's family without being submissive to manipulation.

A happy marriage is built on unity and understanding. Avoid letting family drama interfere with your bond. Address issues early and together.

Boundary Invasion: A Real-Life Scenario

Some families believe invading a couple's privacy is love. A husband or wife may be afraid to confront this intrusion, fearing accusations of disloyalty or drama. Thus, the burden is left on the spouse to endure attacks from in-laws—verbal, emotional, or psychological.

In some cases, husbands excuse themselves from confrontation, saying, "It's between you women." Whether it's slander in his presence or snide remarks behind his back, it's his responsibility to shield his spouse. Sadly, many choose the path of least resistance.

"For this reason a man shall leave his father and mother and be joined to his wife, and the two shall become one flesh." Ephesians 5:31 NKJV

No spouse should stand alone against their in-laws. Marriage is a covenant of unity, not isolation.

What You Can Do

If you're experiencing tension with your in-laws, the most powerful starting point is to focus your energy on improving your relationship with your spouse. Openly express your concerns. Tell him or her, "I want to understand what's truly making your family uncomfortable with me." But assert that you want to speak to them directly—and in your spouse's presence.

Never hold these conversations in your spouse's absence. Doing so invites miscommunication, backbiting, and manipulation. Also, never gather all family members at once for such a discussion. This will only lead them to fortify themselves as a group. Even with the best intentions, your spouse may become overwhelmed and inadvertently take their side.

Instead, address each person one-on-one. Your spouse may resist arranging such meetings, out of fear of offending their family or triggering drama. And be warned: even a gentle conversation can turn confrontational. Why? Because you're challenging the dominant person or group to relinquish control. That may feel threatening to them.

Go into the conversation without judgment, but with clarity. Begin by asking, "Have I offended you in any way?" In essence, you are trying to uncover the root of the discomfort in a respectful manner. Ask them directly but gently, "What are three reasons you feel uncomfortable with me?" Often, two of the reasons will be surface-level or defensive; the third may come closer to the truth.

Manage Your Expectations

Open-mindedness means you must not expect them to change. People only change when they choose to—not because you hope they will. A single conversation won't win them over if they didn't like you before. Instead, aim for small, specific changes: maybe calling once a week or agreeing to end phone conversations by 9 PM.

Be polite, but don't try to win their approval with gifts or excessive service. The idea that "you can win people over with love and service" can backfire. If you go down that road, their expectations may become manipulative and unending. You'll finish one task, only for another demand to follow. Set healthy limits.

Examples:

- You will cook, but not serve everyone at separate times.

- You'll retire to your room at a set hour each night.

- You'll attend family events but not subject yourself to emotional abuse.

Set Boundaries Without Ultimatums

Avoid giving your spouse ultimatums like, "Choose between me and your family." That breeds resentment. Instead, say: "I deserve to be treated with respect. I cannot remain where I am consistently disrespected." Assert your emotional boundaries with clarity and maturity.

Tell your spouse how their inaction makes you feel. For example:

- ❖ "When you don't support me, I feel like I don't matter."
- ❖ "It hurts me when your family insults my parents and you say nothing."

Affirm that you respect your spouse's family and expect the same in return.

Ask the Hard Questions

Are you truly happy in this relationship? Can you live with this kind of emotional strain for the rest of your life?

If your in-laws' interference is causing ongoing conflict and your spouse remains passive, you need to decide what you can do for your own peace. Seek professional help. Suggest couples counseling. If your spouse refuses, go alone. Healing begins when you reclaim control over your emotional wellbeing.

Remember: you cannot change others, only yourself. Ask:

i].   Do I want to keep living hurt, angry, or resentful?

ii].   Is this the version of myself I want to remain?

If the answer is no, then stop waiting for others to change. Stop hoping your spouse or their family will see you differently.

Release and Let Go

Once you have respectfully voiced your feelings and asked for clarity, let it go. Accept the reality: if they are unwilling to accept you for who you are, then for your own peace, accept them for who they are—even if they are difficult or bitter people.

No one can help you unless you want to help yourself. And ask yourself honestly: Why should they help you at all?

CHAPTER 3:

The Monster Ravaging Family Values

Divorce is known by many other names: separation, detachment, dissolution, disunion, division, partition, rupture, and split-up. Each term illustrates the painful process and devastating consequences of divorce when it strikes a marriage.

Let us examine some of these synonyms:

- ❖ Separation: The process of creating a gap between two previously connected parts, with each seeking independence.

- ❖ Detachment: The act of removing a part from the whole, leaving it isolated.

- ❖ Dissolution: The breaking down of something unified into fragmented pieces.

- ❖ Disunion: The termination of unity or agreement.

- ❖ Division: Severing a whole into separate entities.

- ❖ Partition: A physical or emotional split into distinct units.

- ❖ Rupture: A violent or painful break.

These definitions paint a vivid picture of what divorce does to a marriage — it tears apart a once unified bond and leaves both individuals broken and scattered.

A. The Divine Nature of Marriage

Marriage is a superior and sacred law that unites two independent individuals — a man and a woman — into one. This divine law is stronger than the bond between parent and child. While the parent-child relationship is emotional and psychological, the marital bond is spiritual. In fact, Scripture states:

"Therefore shall a man leave his father and his mother and shall cleave to his wife, and they shall become one flesh." Genesis 2:24 (NKJV)

This spiritual law is not subject to repeal or dissolution by any mortal authority. Once the marital covenant is established, it is divinely sealed — intended to last for life.

Jesus emphasized this when questioned about divorce:

"Have you not read that He who made them at the beginning 'made them male and female,' and said, 'For this reason a man shall leave his father and mother and be joined to his wife, and the two shall become one flesh'? So then, they are no longer two but one flesh. Therefore, what God has joined together, let no man separate." Matthew 19:4–6 (NKJV)

Jesus clarified that divorce is not part of God's original plan. The only instance where separation might be considered — and even then, controversially — is due to unfaithfulness. Yet even here, He warned against rushing to dissolve what God has joined

B. Divorce: A Legal Action, But a Spiritual Violation

Modern courts issue divorce certificates and dissolve marriages based on irreconcilable differences. However, in the eyes of God, such legal actions do not annul the spiritual covenant. A judge in Alabama once said during a divorce ruling, "According to heaven's registry, both of you are still married." He was simply affirming what Jesus declared:

"And whoever marries her who is divorced commits adultery." Matthew 19:9 (NKJV)

Only death dissolves the marital covenant:

"For a woman who has a husband is bound by the law to her husband as long as he lives. But if the husband dies, she is released from the law of her husband." Romans 7:2 (NKJV)

C. Endurance in Marriage

At the slightest provocation or disagreement, many today rush to dissolve their marriages. Excuses vary from incompatibility to irreconcilable values. But these reasons often reflect a shallow understanding of love.

The Bible clearly defines the nature and character of love:

"Love is patient and kind. Love is not jealous or boastful or proud or rude. It does not demand its own way. It is not irritable, and it keeps no record of being wronged... Love never gives up, never loses faith, is always hopeful, and endures through every circumstance." 1 Corinthians 13:4–7 (NLT)

Love is not a fleeting emotion. It is not something you merely "feel." Emotions are fickle; love is a choice — an intentional act of the will rooted in the character of God. When we love like God, we don't abandon relationships at the first sign of discomfort.

God never stops loving us, even when we are stubborn, rebellious, and unfaithful. His love sees the bigger picture and endures. As believers, we are called to reflect that same kind of enduring, forgiving love in marriage.

"Most important of all, continue to show deep love for each other, for love covers a multitude of sins." 1 Peter 4:8 (NLT)

D. When Love Seems Lost

We often hear words like, "I can't take it anymore," or "Our relationship is beyond repair." But the truth is, most marriages aren't destroyed by monumental failures — they are undone by a slow erosion of patience, understanding, and communication.

Sometimes, all a struggling marriage needs is an honest reassessment and a willingness to change. Pride, unchecked anger, jealousy, and suspicion are poisons to intimacy. Jealousy, in particular, is a sign of insecurity and emotional immaturity. It gives rise to false accusations and destructive patterns of mistrust. Ironically, in trying to protect the marriage, we may be tearing it apart.

E. Don't Create the Monster

Before you label your spouse a "monster," ask yourself: Have I contributed to who they've become? Often, when we accuse our partner of behavior they haven't exhibited, over time they might begin to act exactly how we feared — not because they wanted to, but because they've been unfairly painted into that corner.

This is why patience, communication, and intentional effort are critical. Like caring for a child with special needs, a healthy marriage often requires sacrifice, dedication, and unconditional love. The path to healing lies not in giving up, but in giving more of ourselves with grace.

There is a reason God brought the two of you together. Divorce might look like an easy escape, but it leaves emotional, spiritual, and generational scars. Before you walk away, ask yourself: Have I truly done all I can to restore and nurture what God ordained?

Separation – Mini Divorce

In liberal societies, any perceived infringement on a spouse's rights is often not tolerated. Consequently, divorce is readily granted on the grounds of real or imagined violations of human rights. It is no surprise then that these societies have some of the highest divorce rates in the world.

Unfortunately, this trend is now spreading rapidly across Africa —Nigeria in particular. Statistics show that out of every ten marriages in Nigeria, three are likely to break up before their tenth anniversary. This is alarming and poses a serious threat to the future of the marriage institution unless drastic steps are taken to arrest this trend.

I am a firm believer in human rights and the importance of

respecting personal boundaries. However, I also believe there should be a balance—because "where your rights end is where another person's rights begin." The institution of marriage should not become a battlefield of individualism, where personal rights take precedence over shared responsibilities.

Marriage in Nigeria—and Africa by extension—was once seen as a sacred bond, deeply rooted in permanence and commitment. It was considered un-African to break a marriage covenant. We believed that once married, always married. We embraced not only the sweet moments of marriage but also its challenges. For us, marriage was truly "for better and for worse."

"But Ruth replied, 'Don't ask me to leave you and turn back. I will go wherever you go and live wherever you live. Your people will be my people, and your God will be my God. I will die where you die and will be buried there. May the Lord punish me severely if I allow anything but death to separate us!'" Ruth 1:16-17 NLT

Separation or Divorce: A Flight from Responsibility

Separation or divorce is often an escape route—a quiet admission of defeat in the face of marital challenges. The popular excuse of "irreconcilable differences" is often cited in court, yet these courts were not present during the marriage proposal, nor did they witness the covenant made between the couple.

If you believe you've done your best and still ended up at the edge of separation, I'll challenge that belief: you haven't done enough. In most cases, you've not explored all the available avenues for resolution.

Ask yourself: What exactly have I done to resolve our differences? What role have I played in this conflict? It's easy to see your spouse's faults—but what about yours?

Marriage is a partnership, a give-and-take relationship. It is not about passing blame but about taking responsibility. Most misunderstandings stem from an inability—or refusal—to see things from your partner's perspective.

Let me define misunderstanding as: "The failure to understand or appreciate the other person's point of view regarding an issue." If you always hold on to your perspective as the only valid one, then true understanding can never be achieved. And that's the breeding ground for frequent fights and emotional disconnection.

The Erosion of Spiritual Meaning in Marriage

The increase in divorce rates across the 19th and 20th centuries coincided with the rise of secular ideologies, the liberalization of societal norms, and the waning influence of religion. In many parts of the world, marriage is no longer seen as a sacred covenant before God but as a temporary arrangement based on personal convenience. This has led to what many refer to as the desecration of marriage.

"She has abandoned her husband and ignores the covenant she made before God." Proverbs 2:17 NLT

"Yet you say, 'Why has the Lord abandoned us?' I'll tell you why! Because the Lord witnessed the vows you and your wife made to each other on your wedding day when you were young. But you have dealt treacherously with her; though she is your companion and your wife by covenant." Malachi 2:14 NLT

What Causes Divorce?

In their research paper "Towards Understanding the Reasons for Divorce," Ilene Wolcott and Jody Hughes noted that the dramatic increase in lifetime divorce probability cannot be explained by personal reasons alone. Broader societal changes must also be considered. These include:

1. Affective Reasons

This includes emotional disconnection, communication breakdowns, and incompatibility. Couples often cite reasons like, "we just drifted apart," or "there's no love or trust anymore." Poor communication and changing values are at the heart of such breakdowns.

2. External Pressures

Financial hardship, job-related stress, societal expectations, and family interference often create unbearable tension. Studies show that financial issues contribute significantly to marital breakdowns. Money problems can lead to depression, low self-esteem, and emotional isolation, which can strain the marriage to its breaking point.

3. Abusive Behavior

Physical violence, emotional abuse, and verbal assaults are some of the most common causes of divorce. In modern relationships, people are less tolerant of abuse, and many—especially women—are choosing to walk away rather than remain victims.

4. Personality Traits

Some marriages end due to deep-seated personality flaws, including jealousy, dominance, addiction, immaturity, or lack of emotional intelligence.

Adultery: A Silent Killer of Marriages

A report from the Leadership Newspaper (February 1, 2014) outlined several divorce cases resulting from infidelity. While many couples are reluctant to name adultery as the official reason for their split, deeper investigation often reveals it as a contributing factor.

The truth is—adultery is a destructive act that erodes trust, respect, and intimacy. It's a sign of poor self-control, and though no one is immune to temptation, we all have the responsibility to avoid environments and relationships that make us vulnerable.

"Nevertheless, to avoid sexual immorality, let every man have his own wife, and let every woman have her own husband." 1 Corinthians 7:2 NKJV

However, marriage alone does not cure infidelity. Many married individuals still fall into extramarital affairs. Why? Sometimes it's poor self-discipline, emotional disconnection, or lack of commitment. Some spouses are driven by dissatisfaction, others by unrealistic comparisons fueled by media and fantasy.

It's time to stop blaming external forces and start looking inward. If your marriage is failing, first check your own heart, your own conduct, and your own priorities. Marriages don't thrive on feelings alone—they flourish through love, sacrifice, discipline, and grace.

Marriage is a sacred covenant. When nurtured with respect, forgiveness, and understanding, it can withstand any storm. But when neglected, it becomes vulnerable to every little breeze.

Let us, therefore, rise to protect this divine institution before it crumbles completely under the weight of modern trends

CHAPTER 4:

I Hate Divorce

The rate of divorce continues to rise daily. As reported in Leadership Newspaper on February 1, 2014, an independent investigation by several reporters concluded that the major cause of divorce is adultery. "In the Holy Bible and the Qur'an, adultery is a terrible sin, but today many marriages are being hunted down by this unholy act," the report noted. In more than fifteen divorce proceedings observed across Nigeria, from the north to the south, all the dissolved marriages cited infidelity as the primary cause.

Divorce should never be considered an alternative. God's intention for marriage never included a backdoor. He declared:

"For I hate divorce!" says the Lord, the God of Israel. "It is as cruel as putting on a victim's bloodstained coat," says the Lord Almighty. "So guard yourself; always remain loyal to your wife." Malachi 2:16 NLT

Can we truly claim to walk with God while practicing what He hates? The sooner we eliminate thoughts of escape from our marriage, the sooner we can start building stability and growth within it.

"A house (marriage) is built by wisdom and becomes strong through good sense. Through knowledge its rooms are filled with all sorts of precious riches and valuables." Proverbs 24:3-4 NLT

"Don't use foul or abusive language. Let everything you say be good and helpful, so that your words will be an encouragement to those who hear them." Ephesians 4:29 NLT

God hates divorce, and so should we. The enemy uses divorce to disrupt divine purpose and undermine family values. When Adam sinned, he blamed God for giving him a wife:

"Who told you that you were naked?" the Lord God asked. "Have you eaten the fruit I commanded you not to eat?" "Yes," Adam admitted, "but it was the woman you gave me who brought me the fruit, and I ate it." Genesis 3:11-12 NLT

The Violence of Divorce

A deeper look at Malachi 2:16 reveals:

"...For it covers one's garment with violence." – Malachi 2:16 NLT

The Hebrew word châmâc, translated "violence," denotes the disruption of a divinely established order. Divorce distorts the sacred union of "two becoming one flesh." You cannot go through divorce and emerge unscathed. Ask those who've walked that path —they'll tell you the emotional, spiritual, and even physical toll it takes.

Worse still, the children often suffer the most. Once loving couples, who covered each other's weaknesses, now air their grievances publicly, pointing fingers without acknowledging their faults.

"If you have disputes about such matters (marital issues), why go to outside judges who are not respected by the church? I am saying this to shame you. Isn't there anyone in all the church wise enough to decide these arguments? But instead, one couple sues another—right in front of unbelievers! To have such lawsuits at all is a real defeat for you. Why not just accept the injustice and leave it at that? Why not let yourselves be cheated? But instead, you yourselves are the ones who do wrong and cheat even your own spouse." 1 Corinthians 6:4-8 NLT

Swallowing your pride to preserve your marriage doesn't reduce your worth. It shows maturity. Ego and pride have destroyed many homes. Let go of your pride, and you may save your home from regret.

Creating a Peaceful Home

Recently, my daughter sent me a simple message: "Please call me." Concerned, I quickly returned her call. But instead of a typical request or need—as is common with students—she said something that deeply moved me: "Daddy, thank you for raising us in a peaceful home."

Her words were unexpected and struck a deep chord in me. Curious, I asked her what prompted this reflection. She told me about a neighboring couple who constantly engaged in physical fights. The chaos in that household reminded her of the calm and safety she experienced growing up—and it made her thankful.

Her appreciation made me pause and reflect:

    i.   Do I truly have a peaceful home?

    ii.   What is a peaceful home?

    iii.   Whose responsibility is it to create and maintain one?

    iv.   How did we build the peace we now enjoy in our home?

    v.   And how do we sustain it?

As I thought back to the beginning of our marital journey, I realized that the peace in our home didn't come by accident. It was the result of conscious, collaborative, and consistent effort. Together, my wife and I determined the kind of home we wanted and committed to building it with purpose.

Structures That Birthed a Peaceful Home

We deliberately put in place certain guiding principles that have helped us nurture peace:

➢ Mutual respect, even when opinions differ

➢ The golden rule: Don't do to others what you wouldn't want done to you

➢ Honesty and transparency at all times

➢ No foul language—ever

➢ Emotional self-control, especially in heated moments

➢ Willingness to help, even when it's inconvenient

➢ Seek peace, always pursue what fosters harmony

Jesus said in John 14:27 (NKJV): "Peace I leave with you, My peace I give to you; not as the world gives do I give to you. Let not your heart be troubled, neither let it be afraid."

What a Peaceful Home is Not:

It's important to first debunk some myths:

    a. A peaceful home is not one where there's no disagreement or misunderstanding.

    b. It's not a place where people are silenced, controlled, or suppressed like robots.

    c. It's not a place of fake smiles, shallow coexistence, or emotional distance.

What a Peaceful Home Is:

a) A peaceful home is where differences are managed, and misunderstandings are resolved without damaging each other.

b) It's a haven for emotional safety, where people can be themselves, rest, and recharge.

c) It's where loved ones can vent frustrations and disappointments—and be understood.

d) It's where people prioritize others' well-being, often above their own.

e) It's a space that encourages serenity over strife, focusing on what we love about each other, not just the faults.

Stacy Karen, in her article "Four Steps to a More Peaceful Home", put it perfectly:

"A peaceful home is something many of us long for—a place where relationships are healthy and people are happy. There's no denying that creating a peaceful home takes work. The road to peace is not smooth or easy, but it's worthy!"

Why a Peaceful Home Matters

Most of our days begin and end at home. If that environment is filled with chaos, it affects our mental and emotional well-being. But when home is peaceful, we step into the world with strength and stability.

And yet, many neglect the importance of home peace. We rush through life—hurrying out the door or collapsing on the couch after a long day—without intentionally cultivating peace. But when you realize that a peaceful home means less stress, more joy, and stronger relationships, it becomes clear: the effort is worth it.

Practical Steps to Cultivating Peace at Home

- Tolerate one another's imperfections. Don't nitpick or magnify trivial annoyances.

- Avoid unnecessary arguments. Not every toothpaste cap deserves a war. Talk about issues calmly.

- Be a good roommate. Do small things—like replacing an empty toilet roll—to show you care.

- Celebrate each other's success, no matter how small. Appreciation builds motivation and closeness.

- Remember your love origin story. Reignite that spark often—through dates, memories, or shared dreams.

- Distinguish love from pity. True love is mutual, while pity can create imbalance.

- Reinforce good behavior with praise, not complaints.

- Take breaks together—a vacation, a walk, or even an hour without screens.

- Adjust expectations. Not all relationships are fairy tales. Be realistic and compassionate.

- Practice forgiveness, even when it's hard. It's always worth it.

- Laugh at yourself. A little humility and humor go a long way.

- Take time apart when necessary. Sometimes, space is the healthiest option.

Grow in emotional maturity. As Carl Jung said, "A highly intense emotional reaction often says more about you than about the person you're reacting to."

Final Thoughts

A peaceful home doesn't mean perfection. It means presence, purpose, and partnership. It's a refuge—not from challenges, but from unhealthy conflict. It's a place where grace abounds, where love is lived daily, and where every family member feels safe and valued.

So I ask you today—what are you doing to create a peaceful home

Divorce Antidote

One of the major causes of marital breakdown today is the lack of a sense of security, especially on the part of the wife. When a woman does not feel safe and secure—emotionally, spiritually, socially, or financially—in her husband, she may begin to withdraw. Eventually, she might opt out of the union altogether.

A wife must feel belonged to, loved, and secure in her husband before she can invest her full personality and potential into the success of the marriage. The Scriptures lay great emphasis on the husband's role in creating this security:

"Husbands, love your wives, just as Christ also loved the church and gave Himself for her..." Ephesians 5:25-26 NKJV

Christ's sacrificial love made the Church—His bride—feel eternally secure. Likewise, when a man shows Christ-like love, he creates a home environment where his wife can thrive.

Understanding the Divine Design

No one can fully discover or unleash their potential in a toxic or unfriendly environment. The soil must be conducive for the seed to grow. The foundation of marital success is rooted in understanding the divine counsel found in Ephesians 5:21–23:

    i.   Submitting to one another—mutual humility and honor

    ii.   Wives submitting to their own husbands in all things

    iii.   Husbands loving their wives sacrificially

    iv.   Wives respecting and honoring their husbands

When these God-ordained roles are embraced, most marital frictions can be curtailed.

The Four Pillars of Security Every Husband Must Provide

As the head of the wife (Ephesians 5:23), a man carries immense responsibility. Just like the physical head contains the brain, eyes, ears, and mouth—functions vital for directing and protecting the body—so must a husband provide direction and security to his wife in the following areas:

1. Spiritual Security

A man must be spiritually sensitive, discerning threats in the atmosphere and interceding for his home. This is not optional—it's a divine assignment.

"But the natural man does not receive the things of the Spirit of God... because they are spiritually discerned." 1 Corinthians 2:14 NKJV

Adam failed in this regard by abdicating spiritual leadership to Eve. Rather than protecting her, he stood by passively. Today, many husbands make the same mistake. Even if your wife is more spiritually active, the responsibility to lead spiritually is still yours.

Do not expose your wife to spiritual dangers. Be her covering. Speak life over your home. Lead in prayer and discernment. God has placed you as the watchman of your family.

2. Emotional Security

Women are emotional beings. Their need for love is deeply rooted in emotional connection. When this need is unmet, they become vulnerable.

According to Dr. Gary and Barbara Rosberg in "Five Love Needs of Men and Women," while men prioritize sexual intimacy, women deeply crave emotional intimacy and communication. Your wife longs for reassurance, affirmation, and heartfelt presence. She wants to know she is seen, loved, and emotionally safe. Love is not just affection—it is also attention, correction, presence, and protection.

Men, do not leave your wives emotionally exposed. Be her confidant and anchor. On the other hand, wives should also avoid weaponizing emotions by depriving their husbands of intimacy. Emotional security goes both ways.

3. Social Security

In many cultures, women are marginalized—culturally, economically, and socially. Marriage should be a place of liberation for the woman, not bondage.

What society has denied her, she should regain in her husband—support, value, and identity. Empower her to thrive without being threatened by her success. Protect her from societal oppression, family injustice, and cultural abuse.

"Her husband is her crown and covering." 1 Corinthians 11:6

NKJV

A godly husband must shield his wife from external pressures, including in-laws and unjust traditions that seek to strip her of dignity.

4. Financial Security

"But if anyone does not provide for his own, and especially for those of his household, he has denied the faith and is worse than an unbeliever." 1 Timothy 5:8 NKJV

Financial provision is a divine mandate. While a wife may earn more and support her home, the husband must not abdicate his responsibility. Even if he cannot provide all, he must show effort, initiative, and a desire to lead.

The mouth, as part of the head, feeds the body. Likewise, the husband, as the head, must see to the nourishment and welfare of his household.

❖ Christ gave His all for the Church. Husbands are called to do the same.

Why Many Women Struggle to Submit

Submission becomes difficult when the wife feels unsafe, unloved, or unprotected. However, when a man provides the right security, a woman will naturally and joyfully submit without coercion.

❖ Treat her like a queen, and she will announce you as her king to the world.

Golden Rules for Husbands and Wives

These timeless principles, drawn from Scripture and life experience, are essential in nurturing a godly and healthy marriage:

1. Don't shout at your spouse. A gentle tone preserves peace. (Proverbs 15:1)

2. Don't speak evil of your spouse to others. (Genesis 2:19)

3. Avoid sharing your affection with outsiders. Adultery is destructive. (Matthew 5:28)

4. Never compare your spouse with others. (2 Corinthians 10:12)

5. Be tender and accommodating, not harsh. (Ephesians 4:2)

6. Hide nothing, not even your finances. (Genesis 2:25)

7. Don't criticize her body—she bore your children. (Proverbs 18:22)

8. Her worth is not her appearance. Cherish her. (Ephesians 5:29)

9. Never quarrel in public. Handle issues privately. (Matthew 1:19)

10. Appreciate your spouse—caring for family is sacrificial. (1 Thessalonians 5:18)

11. Appreciate her cooking or his provision. (Proverbs 31:14)

12. Don't place siblings above your spouse. (Genesis 2:24)

13. Invest in your spouse's spiritual growth. (Ephesians 5:26)

14. Pray and study the Bible together. (James 5:16)

15. Enjoy each other's company and laughter. (Ecclesiastes 9:9)

16. Don't use money as a control tool. (1 Peter 3:7)

17. Shield your spouse's weaknesses. (Ephesians 5:30)

18. Honor each other's parents and families. (Matthew 8:14)

19. Keep saying 'I love you.' (Ephesians 5:25)

20. Strive to be like Christ—the perfect example of a spouse. (Romans 8:29)

Final Word

Divorce is not inevitable. With godly understanding, mutual commitment, and the right environment of security and love, marriage can become a safe haven—a place of growth, joy, and intimacy.

Let every man take up his God-given role as protector, provider, and priest of his home. Let every woman find refuge, identity, and joy under the covering of a godly man.

"He who finds a wife finds a good thing and obtains favor from the Lord." Proverbs 18:22 NKJV

CONCLUSION

Marriage is a sacred and delicate institution that requires the highest level of care, commitment, and intentionality. It is not a venture to be handled casually. Every couple must recognize that they are joint stakeholders in this divine covenant—each with a vital role to play in preserving its sanctity.

Whatever sacrifices are necessary to uphold the marriage are worth making. Why? Because when marriage fails, the very foundation of society begins to crumble. The strength of any nation is not measured solely by its economy or military might, but by the health and stability of its families.

Each couple must therefore strive to discover and develop the mechanisms that work uniquely for them. There is no "one-size-fits-all" formula for a successful marriage. Our personalities, backgrounds, values, and environments are all different—and so must our strategies for growth and harmony.

One critical point to note: never compare your marriage to another's. It is both unwise and unfair. What works for one couple may not work for another. What appears successful on the outside may be struggling within. Rather than comparing, invest that energy into understanding your partner, studying your environment, and building a system that strengthens your unique relationship.

"Through wisdom a house is built, and by understanding it is established; by knowledge the rooms are filled with all precious and pleasant riches." Proverbs 24:3–4 NKJV

May God give you the wisdom, understanding, and grace to nurture and sustain your marriage to the glory of His name.

ABOUT THE BOOK

Rekindling Intimacy and Passion in Your Marriage is a heartfelt, Spirit-led guide designed to help couples rediscover love, deepen connection, and restore purpose in their marital journey. Drawing from biblical principles, pastoral insight, and real-life experiences, this book addresses the hidden cracks in marriages that often go unnoticed until it's too late.

In a world where marital breakdown is increasingly common, this book presents time-tested truths and practical wisdom on how to:

- ❖ Build emotional, spiritual, and physical intimacy

- ❖ Understand and fulfill God's blueprint for marriage

- ❖ Handle conflicts with maturity and grace

- ❖ Create a peaceful and nurturing home environment

- ❖ Protect your union from the subtle threats of modern culture

With chapters that explore topics such as communication, forgiveness, security, respect, and divine order in the home, Rekindling Intimacy and Passion in Your Marriage offers tools that will help couples not only survive—but thrive.

Whether you are newly married, struggling, or simply seeking to enrich your relationship, this book provides clear guidance and godly encouragement to help you build a marriage that honors God and blesses generations to come.

"Marriage is more than a contract—it is a covenant. And when rightly handled, it becomes one of the greatest testimonies of

God's love on earth." Pst. Harrison Okechukwu E

ABOUT THE AUTHOR

Pst Harrison Okechukwu E

Pst. Harrison Okechukwu E is a passionate teacher of the Word, marriage counselor, and pastor with a heart for restoring families and strengthening homes. With decades of ministerial experience, he has been a voice of wisdom and hope to couples seeking healing, direction, and intimacy in their marriages. As a committed servant of God, Pastor Harrison has helped many navigate the turbulent waters of marital challenges through biblical counseling, conferences, and faith-based mentorship. His practical approach to teaching God's Word, combined with real-life examples, has made his ministry relatable and transformative. He is the author of several spiritual and motivational works, and he continues to serve in his calling with humility, compassion, and an unwavering desire to see marriages thrive according to God's original design. Pastor Harrison is married and blessed with children. Together with his wife, he embodies the principles he teaches—living proof that when Christ is the center of a home, peace, joy, and intimacy abound. You can connect with Pst. Harrison Okechukwu E via email at harryokey7@gmail.com or Whatsapp: +234-8023418296, +234-7036845512 for speaking engagements, counseling requests, or ministry resources.